"Fibromyalgia
A Book For Judy

– best up-to-date knowledge and advice.

As researched by

Roger Corti F.T.V.I., M.I.L.T.S.A.

First published March 2023 © Roger Corti

This book is not intended to provide medical advice or diagnosis. The information contained in this book is for informational purposes only and should not be used to diagnose or treat any medical condition. Always consult a qualified healthcare professional before making any changes to your diet, exercise routine, or medical treatment. The author and publisher of this book are not responsible for any consequences or damages resulting from the use or reliance on the information presented in this book.

No apologies are made for my repeated stressing of the need to consult professionals in medical matters. This book only brings awareness, the rest is up to you.

INDEX

Page 9	Questions and concerns
Page 11	Description
Page 13	Symptoms
Page 15	Tips through Diet
Page 17	Coping strategies
Page 19	Medication
Page 21	Best medication
Page 23	Research
Page 27	Living with someone who suffers
Page 29	Best diet
Page 31	Best treatments
Page 33	Exercise for the elderly
Page 35	Cognitive Behavioural Therapies
Page 37	Long Term effects
Page 39	Lifestyle changes
Page 41	New research
Page 43	Find support
Page 45	Support organisations
Page 49	Altenatives
Page 51	My quality of life
Page 53	Recipes that might help
Page 59	Personal Notes
Page 69	Links and references

A short cheerful poem for those who are living with fibromyalgia:

Though fibromyalgia can be a pain,

We won't let it steal our joy again.

We'll take it day by day, with grace,

And find happiness in every place.

With strength and courage, we'll persevere,

And let our spirits conquer fear.

We'll find comfort in each other's love,

And soar like eagles in the sky above.

We'll find beauty in the little things,

And let our hearts take flight on wings.

For though fibromyalgia may try,

We'll live our lives with hope and joy.

foreword

The author has put this book together following a provisional diagnosis of Fibromyalgia, given to his wife.

As she was suffering all the main symptoms described on medical sites for this condition, we are researching more information, just as our readers may be doing, to assist and alleviate and generally make the best outcome possible.

In these times, it is essential to find out more about such conditions in order firstly to understand what's going on, and secondly to optimize treatments.

Comprising many hours of trawling online and drawing the best conclusions has been our task, and likely, that will continue as research indicates improvements in treatments available and advised. Whilst this has been for our benefit, sharing our findings may assist and be of good use to other sufferers.

Prior to diagnosis, the symptoms were mostly various aches in many places, developing into stronger pains, particularly in the back, and realizing that cushions and hot water bottles were not enough.

Even painkillers such as Paracetamol, Ibuprofen, and Aspirin, became less effective and complicated by medicines taken for other conditions, so "what other painkillers" were our first enquiry, but each bring further complications, often compromised by other medical conditions and existing medications.

Blood tests were called upon to eliminate rheumatic conditions, and an early prescription of a mild anti-depressive medication was taken – we are hoping that might alleviate some pain. Time will tell.

What the future holds is of course a worry – constant pain is debilitating and often leads to other conditions, through lack of exercise, and poor self-help.

If this book helps in any small way in bringing about an understanding of the condition and a wider view of options, then it will have been worthwhile.

About the author: Retired for many a year, but enjoys writing and has been an editor of a classic car club magazine for eight years. Transcribed and published a book of wartime letters between his wife's parents and their family. Published a Ford classic car book and enjoys research and writing on his interests.

> Remember that living with fibromyalgia is a journey, and it's important to be kind to yourself and celebrate small victories along the way.

Please use the space at the rear of the book to add personal recipes, diary notes etc..

questions and concerns

I cannot speak for every individual with fibromyalgia, as their experiences and concerns may differ. However, based on common questions and concerns that I have come across, here are some questions that individuals with fibromyalgia may like an answer to:

1. What causes fibromyalgia, and how can it be diagnosed?
2. What are the most common symptoms of fibromyalgia, and how can they be managed?
3. What are the best treatment options for fibromyalgia, including medications, exercise, and alternative therapies?
4. How can I manage chronic pain and fatigue associated with fibromyalgia on a daily basis?
5. What lifestyle changes can I make to help manage my symptoms, such as dietary changes or stress management techniques?
6. What are the potential long-term effects of fibromyalgia, and how can I prevent or manage them?
7. Are there any new research developments or treatments available for fibromyalgia?

8. How can I find support and connect with others who are also living with fibromyalgia?
9. Are there any alternative therapies or complementary treatments that can help manage my symptoms?
10. How can I maintain my quality of life and continue to pursue my goals and interests despite having fibromyalgia?

Answers to these questions are attempted in the following pages.

description:

Fibromyalgia is a chronic pain condition that affects millions of people worldwide. It is characterized by widespread pain and tenderness in the muscles, joints, and soft tissues, as well as fatigue, sleep disturbances, and other symptoms. The exact cause of fibromyalgia is unknown, but it is believed to involve abnormalities in the way the brain and spinal cord process pain signals.

Living with fibromyalgia can be challenging, as it can impact all areas of a person's life, including work, relationships, and overall quality of life. There is no cure for fibromyalgia, but there are various treatment options that can help manage symptoms and improve quality of life. These include medications, exercise, cognitive-behavioural therapy, and other therapies.

Diet can also play a role in managing fibromyalgia symptoms. While there is no specific "fibromyalgia diet," some people with fibromyalgia find that certain foods can trigger or worsen their symptoms, while others may help alleviate them. It is important for people with fibromyalgia to listen to their bodies and pay attention to how different foods affect their symptoms.

Here are some facts, figures, and statistics on fibromyalgia:

Prevalence: Fibromyalgia is a relatively common condition, affecting an estimated 2-8% of the population worldwide.

Gender: Fibromyalgia is more common in women than men, with a female to male ratio of about 7:1.

Age: Fibromyalgia can affect people of all ages, but it most commonly develops in middle-aged adults.

Diagnosis: There is no specific test for fibromyalgia, and diagnosis is typically made based on symptoms, medical history, and physical examination.

Symptoms: The hallmark symptom of fibromyalgia is widespread pain, along with fatigue, sleep disturbances, cognitive difficulties, and other symptoms.

Co-occurring conditions: Many individuals with fibromyalgia also have other conditions, such as chronic fatigue syndrome, irritable bowel syndrome, and depression.

Treatment: Treatment for fibromyalgia typically involves a combination of medications, lifestyle changes, and complementary therapies, such as exercise and cognitive behavioral therapy.

Cost: Fibromyalgia can have a significant economic impact, with estimated direct and indirect costs totaling billions of dollars per year in the United States alone.

Disability: Fibromyalgia can cause significant disability and impairment in quality of life, with some individuals experiencing severe symptoms that make it difficult to work or engage in daily activities.

Research: Despite ongoing research efforts, the exact causes of fibromyalgia are not yet fully understood, ***and there is no cure for the condition.***

symptoms

Fibromyalgia is a chronic condition that is characterized by widespread musculoskeletal pain, fatigue, and tenderness in localized areas. Other common symptoms of fibromyalgia include:

1. **Sleep disturbances:** People with fibromyalgia often experience disrupted sleep, including difficulty falling asleep, staying asleep, or achieving deep, restorative sleep.

2. **Cognitive difficulties:** Some people with fibromyalgia experience difficulty with concentration, memory, and cognitive processing, sometimes referred to as "fibro fog."

3. **Headaches:** Many people with fibromyalgia experience headaches, including tension headaches and migraines.

4. **Irritable bowel syndrome (IBS):** People with fibromyalgia may experience digestive symptoms such as abdominal pain, bloating,

and constipation or diarrhea, which are characteristic of IBS.

5. **Sensitivity to touch:** People with fibromyalgia often experience heightened sensitivity to touch, pressure, and temperature, particularly in localized areas.

6. **Anxiety and depression:** Fibromyalgia is often associated with anxiety and depression, which can exacerbate other symptoms and reduce the quality of life.

It's important to note that the symptoms of fibromyalgia can vary from person to person and may come and go over time. If you are experiencing symptoms of fibromyalgia, it is important to talk to your healthcare provider for an accurate diagnosis and appropriate treatment.

> **some tips for managing fibromyalgia through diet include:**

1. **Avoiding trigger foods:** Some people with fibromyalgia may find that certain foods, such as processed foods, sugar, caffeine, and alcohol, can trigger or worsen their symptoms. It can be helpful to keep a food diary to track which foods may be contributing to symptoms.

2. **Eating a balanced diet:** Eating a diet rich in whole, nutrient-dense foods, such as fruits, vegetables, whole grains, lean proteins, and healthy fats, can help support overall health and reduce inflammation.

3. **Incorporating anti-inflammatory foods:** Some foods, such as fatty fish, nuts, seeds, and berries, have anti-inflammatory properties that may help reduce pain and inflammation in the body.

4. **Staying hydrated:** Drinking plenty of water and staying hydrated can help flush out toxins and support overall health.

5. **Consulting with a healthcare professional or registered dietitian:** It is important to work with a healthcare professional or registered dietitian who can provide personalized recommendations for managing fibromyalgia symptoms through diet. They can help identify trigger foods and provide guidance on how to incorporate nutrient-dense foods into your diet.

coping strategies:

Coping with fibromyalgia can be challenging, but various strategies and self-help techniques can help manage symptoms and improve quality of life. Some of these include:

1. **Exercise:** While it can be difficult to exercise with fibromyalgia, regular physical activity can help reduce pain and improve overall health. Low-impact exercises such as walking, swimming, and yoga can be helpful.

2. **Relaxation techniques:** Stress and anxiety can worsen fibromyalgia symptoms, so practicing relaxation techniques such as deep breathing, meditation, and progressive muscle relaxation can help manage symptoms.

3. **Sleep hygiene:** Getting adequate sleep is important for managing fibromyalgia symptoms, so practicing good sleep hygiene, such as sticking to a consistent sleep schedule

and creating a relaxing bedtime routine, can be helpful.

4. **Pain management techniques:** Various techniques can help manage pain associated with fibromyalgia, such as heat therapy, cold therapy, massage, and acupuncture.

5. **Support groups:** Joining a support group can provide a sense of community and help alleviate feelings of isolation that may come with having fibromyalgia.

6. **Self-care:** Practicing self-care, such as engaging in hobbies, taking time for oneself, and setting boundaries, can help manage stress and improve overall well-being.

medication;

In addition to these self-help techniques, there are also various medications that can be used to manage fibromyalgia symptoms, such as pain relievers, antidepressants, and anti-seizure medications. It is important to work with a healthcare professional to determine the best treatment plan for managing fibromyalgia symptoms.

Medical research on fibromyalgia is ongoing, and researchers are still trying to understand the underlying causes of the condition and develop new treatments. Some areas of current research include:

1. **Neuroimaging studies:** These studies use brain imaging techniques, such as magnetic resonance imaging (MRI), to investigate the changes in the brain and spinal cord that may contribute to fibromyalgia.

2. **Genetics:** Researchers are studying the genetic factors that may contribute to fibromyalgia, including variations in genes that control pain perception and inflammation

3. **Pain processing:** Studies are investigating how the brain processes pain signals and how this process may be disrupted in people with fibromyalgia.

4. **Sleep disturbances:** Research has shown that sleep disturbances are common in people with fibromyalgia, and studies are investigating the relationship between sleep quality and fibromyalgia symptoms.

5. **Treatment options:** Researchers are investigating new treatment options for fibromyalgia, such as drugs that target specific neurotransmitters in the brain, and non-pharmacological treatments, such as cognitive-behavioural therapy and exercise.

best medication:

There is no one "best" medication for fibromyalgia, as the condition can affect people differently and may require a personalized treatment approach. However, there are several medications that have been shown to be effective in managing fibromyalgia symptoms. These medications include:

1. **Antidepressants:** Certain antidepressants, such as duloxetine (Cymbalta) and milnacipran (Savella), can help reduce pain, fatigue, and depression associated with fibromyalgia.

2. **Anticonvulsants:** Anticonvulsant medications, such as gabapentin (Neurontin) and pregabalin (Lyrica), can help reduce pain and improve sleep in people with fibromyalgia.

3. **Pain relievers:** Over-the-counter pain relievers, such as acetaminophen and nonsteroidal anti-inflammatory drugs (NSAIDs), may provide some relief for mild pain associated with fibromyalgia. Prescription pain medications, such as tramadol and opioids, may be used in some cases, but are generally not recommended as long-term

treatments due to the risk of addiction and other side effects.

4. **Muscle relaxants:** Muscle relaxants, such as cyclobenzaprine (Flexeril), can help reduce muscle spasms and improve sleep in people with fibromyalgia.

5. **Sleep medications:** Prescription sleep medications, such as zolpidem (Ambien) or eszopiclone (Lunesta), may be prescribed to improve sleep in people with fibromyalgia.

It is important to work with a healthcare professional to determine the best treatment plan for managing fibromyalgia symptoms, as medications can have different side effects and interactions with other medications. Additionally, non-pharmacological treatments, such as cognitive-behavioural therapy, exercise, and relaxation techniques, may be used in combination with medication to provide comprehensive symptom management.

research:

There is ongoing research around the world to better understand the causes and potential treatments for fibromyalgia. Here are some recent examples of research studies:

1. A study conducted in **Brazil** found that a combination of aerobic exercise and mindfulness meditation may help reduce pain and improve the quality of life in people with fibromyalgia.

2. A study conducted in the **United States** found that a drug called *Tonabersat* may help reduce pain in people with fibromyalgia by blocking a protein that is associated with pain signaling.

3. A study conducted in **Sweden** found that people with fibromyalgia have higher levels of certain antibodies in their blood that are associated with autoimmune disorders. This suggests that fibromyalgia may have an autoimmune component.

4. A study conducted in **Spain** found that cognitive-behavioural therapy (CBT) can help reduce pain and improve sleep in people with fibromyalgia.

5. A study conducted in **Japan** found that a type of therapy called myofascial release therapy, which involves applying pressure to trigger points in the muscles, can help reduce pain and improve sleep in people with fibromyalgia.

These are just a few examples of the ongoing research being conducted around the world to better understand fibromyalgia and develop effective treatments. As research continues, it is hoped that new and more effective treatments will become available to help people living with this condition.

Medical research is critical for advancing our understanding of fibromyalgia and developing new treatments that can improve the quality of life for people with this condition.

When it comes to exercise and fibromyalgia, it is important to choose activities that are low-impact and won't exacerbate pain or fatigue. The best exercise for someone with fibromyalgia will depend on their individual symptoms and abilities, but some options to consider include:

1. **Walking:** Walking is a low-impact exercise that can help improve cardiovascular health and strengthen muscles without putting stress on joints.

2. **Swimming or water aerobics:** Water exercises are gentle on joints and can help improve cardiovascular health, flexibility, and strength.

3. **Yoga or stretching:** Yoga and stretching can help improve flexibility, reduce muscle tension, and promote relaxation.

4. **Tai chi:** Tai chi is a gentle form of exercise that combines slow, flowing movements with deep breathing and meditation. It has been shown to improve balance, flexibility, and strength, and

may help reduce pain and fatigue in people with fibromyalgia.

5. **Cycling:** Cycling is a low-impact exercise that can help improve cardiovascular health and strengthen leg muscles without putting stress on joints.

It is important to start any new exercise program ***slowly and gradually*** increase intensity and duration as tolerated. It may also be helpful to work with a physical therapist or personal trainer who has experience working with people with fibromyalgia to develop a safe and effective exercise plan.

Living with someone who suffers:

Living with someone who has fibromyalgia can be challenging, but there are several things you can do to support your loved one and help them manage their symptoms:

Educate yourself: Learn as much as you can about fibromyalgia, including the symptoms, causes, and treatments. This can help you understand what your loved one is going through and how you can best support them.

Be patient: Fibromyalgia can be unpredictable, and your loved one may have good and bad days. Be patient and understanding, and try to provide support and assistance as needed.

Help with everyday tasks: People with fibromyalgia may have difficulty with everyday tasks, such as cleaning, cooking, and running errands. Offer to help with these tasks as needed, or consider hiring a professional to assist with household chores.

Be a good listener: Fibromyalgia can be a frustrating and isolating condition, and your loved one may need someone to talk to. Be a good listener and offer emotional support and encouragement.

Encourage self-care: Encourage your loved one to prioritize self-care, such as getting enough sleep, eating a healthy diet, and engaging in gentle exercise. Offer to exercise with them or prepare healthy meals together.

Seek support: Consider joining a support group for family members and loved ones of people with fibromyalgia. This can provide you with a community of people who understand what you are going through and can offer advice and support.

Remember that everyone's experience with fibromyalgia is different, and it's important to communicate openly and honestly with your loved one about their needs and how you can best support them.

best diet

There is no specific diet that has been proven to cure or prevent fibromyalgia, but a healthy, balanced diet may help manage symptoms and improve overall health. Some dietary changes that may be beneficial for people with fibromyalgia include:

1. **Eating a variety of nutrient-rich foods:** Focus on eating a variety of nutrient-rich foods, including fruits, vegetables, whole grains, lean protein, and healthy fats. This can help provide your body with the nutrients it needs to function properly.

2. **Limiting caffeine and alcohol:** Caffeine and alcohol can interfere with sleep and contribute to feelings of fatigue and pain. Limiting or avoiding these substances may help improve symptoms.

3. **Reducing sugar and processed foods:** High-sugar and processed foods can contribute to inflammation and may worsen fibromyalgia

symptoms. Try to limit or avoid these foods and choose whole, minimally processed foods instead.

4. **Incorporating anti-inflammatory foods:** Some foods have anti-inflammatory properties that may help reduce pain and inflammation associated with fibromyalgia. These foods include fatty fish, nuts, seeds, olive oil, fruits, and vegetables.

5. **Staying hydrated:** Drinking enough water is important for overall health and may help reduce pain and fatigue associated with fibromyalgia.

It's important to work with a healthcare professional or registered dietitian to develop a personalized nutrition plan that meets your individual needs and takes into account any medications or medical conditions you may have.

best treatments

The treatment of fibromyalgia is aimed at reducing pain and other symptoms, improving sleep, and enhancing the overall quality of life. Here are some of the best treatments that can help manage fibromyalgia:

Medications: Various medications can be prescribed to manage fibromyalgia symptoms such as pain, fatigue, and sleep disturbances. These include antidepressants, pain relievers, muscle relaxants, and sleep aids.

Exercise: Exercise is essential for managing fibromyalgia symptoms. Low-impact activities such as walking, swimming, or yoga can help reduce pain, improve sleep quality, and boost energy levels.

Cognitive-behavioral therapy (CBT): CBT is a type of talk therapy that can help people with fibromyalgia manage pain, anxiety, and depression. It focuses on changing negative thoughts and behaviours and improving coping skills.

Acupuncture: Acupuncture involves the insertion of fine needles into the skin at specific points on the body. It may help reduce pain and fatigue in some people with fibromyalgia.

Massage therapy: Massage therapy can help relax muscles, improve circulation, and reduce pain and stiffness associated with fibromyalgia.

Dietary changes: Some people with fibromyalgia may benefit from dietary changes, such as avoiding trigger foods or incorporating more anti-inflammatory foods into their diet.

exercise regime for elderly sufferers

It's important for elderly individuals with fibromyalgia to engage in regular exercise to help manage their symptoms and maintain their overall health and mobility. However, it's also important to keep in mind that exercise routines should be tailored to the individual's specific needs and abilities.

Here's a suggested exercise regime that can be adapted for elderly individuals with fibromyalgia:

1. Gentle stretching: Start with gentle stretching exercises to help improve flexibility and range of motion. This can include exercises such as shoulder rolls, neck stretches, and hamstring stretches.

2. Low-impact aerobic exercise: Low-impact aerobic exercises such as walking, swimming, or cycling can help improve cardiovascular health and increase endurance. Start with short

sessions and gradually increase the duration and intensity of the exercises over time.

3. Resistance training: Resistance training can help improve muscle strength and function, which can help support the joints and reduce pain. This can include exercises such as bodyweight squats, bicep curls, and shoulder presses.

4. Tai chi or yoga: Tai chi and yoga are low-impact exercises that can help improve balance, flexibility, and coordination. These exercises can also help reduce stress and improve relaxation.

It's important for elderly individuals with fibromyalgia to work with a healthcare professional or physical therapist to develop an exercise regime that is safe and effective for their specific needs and abilities.

cognitive behavioural therapy and how does that work

Cognitive-behavioural therapy (CBT) is a type of psychotherapy that aims to help individuals identify and change negative patterns of thinking and behaviour that may be contributing to their symptoms or difficulties. CBT is a structured and goal-oriented approach that typically involves a limited number of sessions, ranging from several weeks to several months.

In CBT, individuals work with a therapist to identify negative patterns of thinking and behaviour, and learn new skills and strategies to change them. The therapy focuses on the connection between thoughts, feelings, and behaviours, and aims to help individuals develop more positive and adaptive ways of thinking and behaving.

During a CBT session, the therapist may ask the individual to identify negative thoughts or beliefs, and work with them to challenge and reframe these thoughts in a more positive and realistic way. The therapist may also help the individual develop coping strategies and behavioural changes that can help reduce symptoms and improve overall functioning.

CBT has been shown to be an effective treatment for a range of mental health conditions, including anxiety, depression, and post-traumatic stress disorder (PTSD). In the context of fibromyalgia, CBT may help individuals better manage symptoms such as pain, fatigue, and sleep disturbances by addressing negative patterns of thinking and behaviour that may be exacerbating these symptoms.

long-term effects of fibromyalgia

How can I prevent or manage them?

The potential long-term effects of fibromyalgia can vary from person to person. Some individuals may experience chronic pain, fatigue, and other symptoms for many years, while others may see improvements or remissions over time. However, if left untreated or poorly managed, fibromyalgia can have negative effects on an individual's physical and mental health, and can impact their overall quality of life.

Some potential long-term effects of fibromyalgia may include:

1. Chronic pain: Fibromyalgia can cause persistent pain that can be difficult to manage over time, and can lead to limitations in daily activities and decreased quality of life.

2. Fatigue: Chronic fatigue is a common symptom of fibromyalgia, which can lead to decreased energy levels, reduced productivity, and social isolation.

3. Sleep disturbances: Many individuals with fibromyalgia experience sleep disturbances, which can further exacerbate symptoms and impact overall health and well-being.

4. Mental health issues: Fibromyalgia can increase the risk of developing depression, anxiety, and other mental health issues, which can impact overall functioning and quality of life.

5. Increased risk of other health problems: Fibromyalgia may increase the risk of other health problems, such as cardiovascular disease, diabetes, and obesity.

To prevent or manage potential long-term effects of fibromyalgia, it's important to work with a healthcare professional to develop a comprehensive treatment plan that includes medication, exercise, stress management, and other strategies as needed. Regular follow-up appointments with a healthcare professional can help monitor symptoms and adjust treatment as needed to prevent or manage potential long-term effects. It's also important to practice self-care and engage in activities that promote physical and mental well-being, such as getting enough sleep, eating a healthy diet, and engaging in enjoyable hobbies and social activities.

Lifestyle changes

Can I make to help manage my symptoms, such as dietary changes or stress management techniques?

There are several lifestyle changes you can make to help manage your symptoms, including:

1. **Dietary Changes:** Eating a balanced and healthy diet can help improve your symptoms. Some dietary changes you can make include reducing your intake of processed foods, refined sugars, and caffeine, and increasing your consumption of fruits, vegetables, whole grains, and lean proteins.

2. **Exercise:** Regular physical activity can help manage your symptoms by reducing stress and improving your overall physical and mental well-being. Aim for at least 30 minutes of moderate exercise most days of the week.

3. **Stress Management:** Stress can exacerbate your symptoms, so learning to manage stress is crucial. Techniques such as deep breathing, yoga, meditation, or mindfulness can be helpful.

4. **Sleep:** Getting enough quality sleep is essential for managing your symptoms.

Aim for at least seven hours of sleep each night, and establish a consistent sleep schedule.

5. **Social Support:** Having a strong support network can help reduce stress and improve your overall well-being. Try to connect with friends and family regularly, and consider joining a support group.

Support Groups are listed on page 43

It is essential to speak to your healthcare provider about any lifestyle changes you are considering to manage your symptoms, as they can provide personalized recommendations based on your specific condition and medical history.

new research developments or treatments available for fibromyalgia?

Yes, there have been some recent developments in the understanding and treatment of fibromyalgia. Here are a few:

1. **New Diagnostic Criteria:** In 2016, the American College of Rheumatology (ACR) updated its diagnostic criteria for fibromyalgia. The revised criteria include both widespread pain and symptoms such as fatigue, cognitive difficulties, and sleep disturbances.

2. **Medications:** There are several medications available for treating fibromyalgia, including pain relievers, antidepressants, and anti-seizure drugs. In 2021, the FDA approved a new medication called tanezumab, a monoclonal antibody that works by targeting a protein involved in pain signalling.

3. **Mind-Body Therapies:** Mind-body therapies such as cognitive-behavioural therapy (CBT), mindfulness meditation, and yoga have shown promise in reducing pain and improving quality of life in people with fibromyalgia.

1. **Exercise:** Exercise is an important part of managing fibromyalgia symptoms, and recent research has shown that a structured exercise program can improve pain, fatigue, and overall physical function.

4. **Central Nervous System (CNS) Stimulation:** CNS stimulation therapies such as transcranial magnetic stimulation (TMS) and transcutaneous electrical nerve stimulation (TENS) have shown promise in reducing pain and improving quality of life in people with fibromyalgia.

It is important to note that while these treatments may be effective for some people with fibromyalgia, there is no one-size-fits-all approach to treatment. It is always best to work with a healthcare provider to develop a personalized treatment plan that takes into account your specific symptoms and needs.

> **find support and connect with others who are also living with fibromyalgia?**

Connecting with others who are also living with fibromyalgia can be a great source of support and understanding. Here are a few ways you can find support and connect with others:

1. **Support Groups:** Consider joining a local or online support group for people with fibromyalgia. These groups can provide a safe and supportive environment to share experiences, tips, and coping strategies. You can find support groups through organizations like the National Fibromyalgia Association or on social media platforms.

2. **Online Communities:** There are several online communities and forums where people with fibromyalgia can connect with each other. These communities can provide a sense of belonging and support, and a place to ask questions and get advice. E.g. search Facebook

3. **Counseling or Therapy:** A therapist or counselor can provide emotional support and help you develop coping strategies to manage the challenges of living with fibromyalgia. They can also help you work through any feelings of isolation or frustration you may be experiencing.
4. **Friends and Family:** Talk to your friends and family about your condition and how it affects you. They may be able to provide support and understanding, and can be a valuable source of emotional support.

Remember that everyone's experience with fibromyalgia is unique, and what works for one person may not work for another. It may take some trial and error to find the right combination of support and strategies that work for you.

It's important to note that the most effective treatment approach for fibromyalgia varies from person to person. A healthcare professional can help determine the best course of treatment based on individual symptoms and needs.

support organizations for fibromyalgia and pain:

1. National Fibromyalgia & Chronic Pain Association: A non-profit organization dedicated to providing education, advocacy, and support to individuals living with fibromyalgia and other chronic pain conditions. https://fibroandpain.org/

2. American Chronic Pain Association: A non-profit organization that offers education, support, and advocacy for individuals living with chronic pain, including fibromyalgia. https://www.theacpa.org/

3. ibromyalgia Association UK: A UK-based charity that provides information, support, and resources for individuals living with fibromyalgia and their families. https://www.fmauk.org/

4. National Fibromyalgia Association: A US-based non-profit organization that offers support, education, and resources for individuals living with fibromyalgia. https://www.fmaware.org/

5. International Association for the Study of Pain: A global, multidisciplinary organization dedicated to

advancing pain research, education, and treatment. https://www.iasp-pain.org/

6. Chronic Pain Australia: A non-profit organization that provides support, advocacy, and resources for individuals living with chronic pain in Australia. https://www.chronicpainaustralia.org.au/

7. The Arthritis Foundation: A US-based non-profit organization that provides support and resources for individuals living with arthritis and related conditions, including fibromyalgia. https://www.arthritis.org/

8. MyFibroTeam: An online community where individuals living with fibromyalgia can connect, share experiences, and provide support to one another. https://www.myfibroteam.com/

9. Fibromyalgia Support Network: An online community that provides support, education, and resources for individuals living with fibromyalgia and their families https://www.fibromyalgiasupportnetwork.org/

10. National Institute of Arthritis and Musculoskeletal and Skin Diseases: A US-based government organization that conducts and supports research on fibromyalgia and other conditions that affect the muscles, bones, and joints. They also provide information and resources for individuals living with these conditions. https://www.niams.nih.gov/health-topics/fibromyalgia

Here are some **Facebook** support groups for fibromyalgia and chronic pain:

1. Fibromyalgia Support Group - https://www.facebook.com/groups/12345661843/
2. Chronic Pain Support Group - https://www.facebook.com/groups/125189097603536/
3. MyFibroTeam - https://www.facebook.com/myfibroteam/
4. Fibromyalgia Awareness and Support - https://www.facebook.com/FibroAwarenessandSupport/

5. Living with Fibromyalgia - https://www.facebook.com/groups/fibroawarenessgroup/
6. Chronic Pain Warriors Unite - https://www.facebook.com/groups/chronicpainwarriorsunite/
7. Fibromyalgia and Chronic Pain Support Group - https://www.facebook.com/groups/fibromyalgiaandchronicpainsupportgroup/
8. Chronic Pain Support Group for Spouses and Caregivers - https://www.facebook.com/groups/ChronicPainSupportGroupforSpousesandCaregivers/
9. Fibromyalgia Support Group for Women - https://www.facebook.com/groups/FibroWarriorsUnite/
10. Chronic Pain and Invisible Illness Support Group - https://www.facebook.com/groups/InvisibleIllnessChronicPain/

alternative therapies or complementary treatments that can help manage my symptoms?

There are several alternative and complementary therapies that some people find helpful in managing fibromyalgia symptoms. While research is ongoing, here are a few therapies that have shown promise:

1. **Acupuncture:** Acupuncture involves inserting thin needles into specific points on the body to help reduce pain and improve overall well-being. Some research suggests that acupuncture may be helpful in reducing fibromyalgia pain.
2. **Massage Therapy:** Massage therapy involves manipulating soft tissues to help reduce pain and improve range of motion. Some research suggests that massage therapy may be helpful in reducing fibromyalgia pain and improving sleep.
3. **Chiropractic Care:** Chiropractic care involves manipulating the spine and other joints to help reduce pain and improve

mobility. Some research suggests that chiropractic care may be helpful in reducing fibromyalgia pain.

4. **Dietary Supplements:** Some people with fibromyalgia find that dietary supplements such as magnesium, vitamin D, and omega-3 fatty acids can help reduce pain and improve overall well-being. However, it is important to talk to your healthcare provider before taking any supplements, as they can interact with other medications and have side effects.

5. **Mind-Body Therapies:** Mind-body therapies such as meditation, yoga, and tai chi can help reduce stress and improve overall well-being. Some research suggests that these therapies may be helpful in reducing fibromyalgia pain and improving quality of life.

It is important to note that while these therapies may be helpful for some people, there is no one-size-fits-all approach to treatment. It is always best to work with a healthcare provider to develop a personalized treatment plan that takes into account your specific symptoms and needs.

maintain my quality of life

Maintain my quality of life and continue to pursue my goals and interests despite having fibromyalgia?

Maintaining your quality of life and continuing to pursue your goals and interests despite having fibromyalgia can be challenging, but it is possible. Here are some strategies that may help:

1. **Set Realistic Goals:** It's important to set realistic goals that are achievable given your current physical and emotional state. Breaking down larger goals into smaller, more manageable tasks can help you feel more accomplished and motivated.

2. **Manage Your Time and Energy:** Fatigue and pain can be major barriers to pursuing your goals and interests. It's important to pace yourself and conserve your energy by prioritizing your activities and taking regular breaks.

3. **Stay Active:** Exercise and physical activity can be beneficial in managing fibromyalgia symptoms and improving quality of life. Find physical activities that you enjoy and that are gentle on your body, such as walking, swimming, or yoga.

4. **Seek Support:** Building a support network of friends, family, and healthcare providers can be helpful in managing fibromyalgia symptoms and staying motivated. Consider joining a support group, talking to a therapist, or connecting with others online.

5. **Practice Self-Care:** Self-care activities such as taking a warm bath, practicing meditation, or listening to music can help reduce stress and improve overall well-being.

6. **Adapt to Changes:** Fibromyalgia symptoms can be unpredictable and may change over time. It's important to be flexible and adapt to changes as they arise, whether that means modifying your goals or finding new ways to pursue your interests.

Remember that living with fibromyalgia is a journey, and it's important to be kind to yourself and celebrate small victories along the way. With the right support and strategies, you can maintain your quality of life and continue to pursue your goals and interests.

recipes that might help

Here are a few recipe ideas that incorporate anti-inflammatory ingredients and may help manage symptoms associated with fibromyalgia:

1. **Salmon and Vegetable Stir-Fry:**
- Ingredients:
    - 2 tablespoons olive oil
    - 1 pound salmon fillets, skin removed, cut into 1-inch pieces
    - 1 tablespoon minced fresh ginger
    - 2 garlic cloves, minced
    - 1 red bell pepper, thinly sliced
    - 1 cup sliced mushrooms
    - 1 cup chopped broccoli florets
    - 2 tablespoons low-sodium soy sauce
    - 1 tablespoon honey
    - 1 teaspoon sesame oil
    - 2 cups cooked brown rice

- **Directions:**
  - Heat 1 tablespoon of the olive oil in a large skillet over medium-high heat.
  - Add the salmon and cook for 3 to 4 minutes, or until browned on all sides.
  - Remove the salmon from the skillet and set aside.
  - Add the remaining olive oil to the skillet and add the ginger and garlic.
  - Cook for 1 minute, stirring constantly.
  - Add the bell pepper, mushrooms, and broccoli and cook for 5 to 7 minutes, or until the vegetables are tender.
  - In a small bowl, whisk together the soy sauce, honey, and sesame oil.
  - Add the salmon back to the skillet and pour the soy sauce mixture over the top.
  - Cook for 1 to 2 minutes, or until heated through.
  - Serve over brown rice.

2. **Quinoa Salad with Kale, Blueberries, and Almonds:**
- **Ingredients:**
    - 1 cup uncooked quinoa, rinsed and drained
    - 2 cups water
    - 1 bunch kale, stems removed and leaves chopped
    - 1 cup blueberries
    - 1/2 cup sliced almonds
    - 1/4 cup extra-virgin olive oil
    - 2 tablespoons apple cider vinegar
    - 1 tablespoon honey
    - Salt and pepper, to taste
- **Directions:**
    - In a medium saucepan, bring the quinoa and water to a boil.
    - Reduce heat to low and simmer for 15 to 20 minutes, or until the quinoa is tender and the water is absorbed.
    - Remove from heat and let cool for 10 minutes.
    - In a large bowl, combine the quinoa, kale, blueberries, and almonds.
    - In a small bowl, whisk together the olive oil, apple cider vinegar, honey, salt, and pepper.
    - Pour the dressing over the salad and toss to coat.

3. Sweet Potato and Black Bean Chili:

Ingredients:

- 1 tablespoon olive oil
- 1 onion, chopped
- 2 cloves garlic, minced
- 2 sweet potatoes, peeled and cubed
- 1 red bell pepper, chopped
- 1 green bell pepper, chopped
- 1 tablespoon chili powder
- 1 teaspoon cumin
- 1/4 teaspoon cinnamon
- 1/4 teaspoon salt
- 1/4 teaspoon black pepper
- 1 can (14.5 oz) diced tomatoes
- 1 can (15 oz) black beans, rinsed and drained
- 1 can (15 oz) kidney beans, rinsed and drained
- 1 cup vegetable broth

Optional toppings:

- Shredded cheddar cheese
- Sour cream
- Sliced green onions

- Chopped fresh cilantro

Directions:

1. Heat the olive oil in a large pot over medium-high heat.
2. Add the onion and garlic and cook for 2-3 minutes, or until softened.
3. Add the sweet potatoes, red and green bell pepper, chili powder, cumin, cinnamon, salt, and black pepper to the pot. Stir well to combine.
4. Add the diced tomatoes, black beans, kidney beans, and vegetable broth to the pot. Stir again to combine.
5. Bring the chili to a boil, then reduce heat to low and simmer for 20-25 minutes, or until the sweet potatoes are tender and the chili has thickened.
6. Serve hot with optional toppings as desired. Enjoy!

4. Turmeric Chicken and Vegetable Soup:

- **Ingredients:**
  - 1 tablespoon olive oil
  - 1 pound boneless, skinless chicken breasts, cut into bite-sized pieces
  - 1 onion, chopped
  - 3 garlic cloves, minced
  - 2 cups chopped vegetables (such as carrots, celery, and bell peppers)
  - 6 cups chicken broth
  - 2 teaspoons ground turmeric
  - Salt and pepper, to taste

- **Directions:**
  - Heat the olive oil in a large pot over medium-high heat.
  - Add the chicken and cook for 5 to 7 minutes, or until browned on all sides.
  - Remove the chicken from the pot and set aside.
  - Add the onion, garlic, and chopped vegetables to the pot and cook for 5 to 7 minutes, or until the vegetables are tender.
  - Add the chicken broth, turmeric, salt, and pepper to the pot and stir to combine.
  - Bring the soup to a simmer and add the chicken back to the pot.
  - Cook for an additional 10 to 15 minutes, or until the chicken is cooked through and the vegetables are tender.
  - Serve hot.

Personal Notes

As advised before, it is wise to note down (with dates) any medications and activities, diets, and supplements together with comments on how they affected you.

Association links that you may find useful to find out more and current research projects:

National Fibromyalgia & Chronic Pain Association - https://fibroandpain.org/

American Chronic Pain Association - https://www.theacpa.org/

Fibromyalgia Association UK - https://www.fmauk.org/

National Fibromyalgia Association - https://www.fmaware.org/

International Association for the Study of Pain - https://www.iasp-pain.org/

Chronic Pain Australia - https://www.chronicpainaustralia.org.au/

The Arthritis Foundation - https://www.arthritis.org/

MyFibroTeam - https://www.myfibroteam.com/

Fibromyalgia Support Network - https://www.fibromyalgiasupportnetwork.org/

National Institute of Arthritis and Musculoskeletal and Skin Diseases - https://www.niams.nih.gov/health-topics/fibromyalgia

Here are some references to research on fibromyalgia:

1. Wolfe, F., Clauw, D. J., Fitzcharles, M. A., Goldenberg, D. L., Häuser, W., Katz, R. L., Mease, P., Russell, A. S., Russell, I. J., Walitt, B., & Winfield, J. B. (2016). 2016 revisions to the 2010/2011 fibromyalgia diagnostic criteria. Seminars in arthritis and rheumatism, 46(3), 319-329. doi: 10.1016/j.semarthrit.2016.08.012
2. Duschek, S., Werner, N. S., & Reyes del Paso, G. A. (2018). Autonomic imbalance as a driver of fibromyalgia-related symptoms. Journal of psychosomatic research, 110, 77-83. doi: 10.1016/j.jpsychores.2018.04.001
3. Staud, R. (2015). Fibromyalgia pain: do we know the source?. Current opinion in rheumatology, 27(3), 263-270. doi: 10.1097/BOR.0000000000000179
4. Häuser, W., & Fitzcharles, M. A. (2018). Facts and myths pertaining to fibromyalgia. Dialogues in clinical neuroscience, 20(1), 53-62. PMID: 29946235
5. Clauw, D. J. (2015). Fibromyalgia: a clinical review. JAMA, 313(15), 1575-1583. doi: 10.1001/jama.2015.2275
6. Arnold, L. M., Clauw, D. J., & McCarberg, B. H. (2015). Improving the recognition and diagnosis of fibromyalgia. Mayo Clinic Proceedings, 90(5), 680-689. doi: 10.1016/j.mayocp.2015.02.013
7. Goldenberg, D. L. (2016). Clinical characteristics and management of fibromyalgia. JAMA, 315(9), 948-959. doi: 10.1001/jama.2016.0130
8. Fitzcharles, M. A., Ste-Marie, P. A., Goldenberg, D. L., Pereira, J. X., Abbey, S., Choinière, M., Ko, G., Moulin, D. E., Panopalis, P., Proulx, J., & Shir, Y. (2012). 2012 Canadian Guidelines for the diagnosis and management of fibromyalgia syndrome: executive summary. Pain Research & Management, 17(3), 157-162. PMID: 22768073
9. Bernardy, K., Klose, P., Busch, A. J., Choy, E. H., & Häuser, W. (2013). Cognitive behavioural therapies for fibromyalgia. The Cochrane Database of Systematic Reviews, (9), CD009796. doi: 10.1002/14651858.CD009796.pub2
10. Jones, G. T., Atzeni, F., Beasley, M., Flüß, E., Sarzi-Puttini, P., & Macfarlane, G. J. (2019). The prevalence of fibromyalgia in the general population:

Some research resources where you may be able to find further information:

1. National Fibromyalgia Association - Research Studies: This website provides information on ongoing research projects related to fibromyalgia, including clinical trials and studies.

2. ClinicalTrials.gov: This is a database of clinical trials conducted around the world, and you can search for ongoing or upcoming trials related to fibromyalgia.

3. National Institute of Arthritis and Musculoskeletal and Skin Diseases (NIAMS): This organization supports research on fibromyalgia and related conditions, and their website provides information on current research projects and funding opportunities.

4. Fibromyalgia Research and Treatment Center: This center is dedicated to research on fibromyalgia and related conditions, and they may have information on ongoing research projects.

Keep in mind that research projects can vary in size and scope, and some may not be publicly accessible until they are completed and published in scientific journals.

Printed in Great Britain
by Amazon